CONTENTS

	Page
1. Against all Odds	5
2. A teacher's lesson	10
3. Story of my sisters	15
4. Help yourself	21
5. Fighter's story	25
6. Dance with Life	32
7. Mother who could not be a role model	39
8. Truth of many a women	42
9. For others it's like a story	46
10. Move on	52
11. Agents of change	57

DEDICATION

This book is dedicated to all the women.Some scared, some angry, some shy, some depressed, but above all brave enough to share a part of them with the outside judgemental world so that others become wiser.

ACKNOWLEDGEMENT

I would like to thank the almighty for showing me the way and giving me the strength to work with women on breast cancer awareness. I own a humble thanks to all those people who came along the way, be it patients, their families or friends to share their stories and emotions with me, some personal and some not so personal. I sincerely acknowledge the efforts of women who motivated me to write their stories.

PREFACE

This compilation was motivated by the zeal and enthusiasm of some of the women undergoing treatment for breast cancer who wanted to reach out to many more like them and help them in whatever way possible.

Breast cancer happens to be the commonest form of cancer amongst women from India but most of the women come to the hospital only when the disease has reached the advanced stage. The author has been conducting breast health awareness workshops in India for more than a decade now and has been empowering women to detect the disease at the earliest.

The stories have been written in simple language, verbatim have been incorporated wherever appropriate. Name of the characters have been changed to maintain confidentiality of the women and permission has been taken from them to compile their stories. This endeavour aims at making the stories from India available to all as issues of women regarding health from across the globe have a lot in common.

STORY 1

AGAINST ALL ODDS

Kusum was not sure of her age, maybe she was 27 or 28 years old. She was operated for breast cancer ten months back. Six cycles of chemotherapy were already given and now she was waiting for radiation therapy to start. She lived in Haryana before her marriage. Got married at about 17 or 18 and then moved to Delhi. Her husband had a small electrical parts shop and she was a fulltime housewife. Her mother in law also lived with them.She was a teacher at a primary level government school. Kusum had three sons, elder was 8 years, and then 4 and 3 years. She had three children.....all sons a cause of envy for a number of women from not only rural background like her but also urban. She would manage the whole house from morning till late night again to get up early next day to repeat the cycle. She barely spoke to anyone from outside of the house as her mother in law was against it and Kusum was too busy to bother.

One day while washing clothes she got wet and touched her right breast to feel how much wet her *kurta* had become that she felt a small lump about the size of a small tiny grain. She could feel it with her fingers clearly and it would slide under her fingers easily. She told about it to her mother in law. Mother in law advised Kusum not to bother as according to her it was just a milk gland and many women this kind of harmless lump. Kusum told her that she had stopped breast feeding 2 years back and it was not likely to be a lump related to milk secretion. Her mother in laws friends who visited them once in a while also told her the same. She thought to herself had the lump been painful and she cried about it and made noise her husband would have taken her to the doctor.

Time passed and the lump increased in size. At the back of her mind she was scared it could be something serious. She no longer wanted to ignore the increase in size. She grew anxious by the day as to what that lump could be. A few more months elapsed and she gathered the courage to ask her husband to take her to a nearby government health centre. The doctors over there immediately asked her to go to a hospital where she could be investigated thoroughly. By now her lump had increased to the size of a small ball which on pressing was still painless. Her husband within a week took her to a speciality hospital through a friend of his who worked there in a lab. Kusum was investigated within a weeks' time. She was in stage II of breast cancer. Had her husband not know the staff of this hospital it would have taken her a few more months to get investigated. However for surgery they had to wait longer as no beds were available. She was discharged after the surgery and told to do exercises for my arm. She did not know what to say about side effects of surgery or 6 cycles of chemotherapy that followed.... She had three sons and they had to be looked after. Her husband would leave for work at 8 in the morning to return back home only at 11at night. Mother in law would go to school early in the morning and come back in the afternoon. Kusum had to cook, clean, walk the children to school, wash clothes, utensils, make her sons do homework and cook again. She had no help at home and did not know how the day passed. She didn't have time to think about what to eat and when, forget about the special diet and rest .She felt fatigued and sick at times but had no choice. This was her daily routine ever since she got married to … surgery … to chemotherapy…. and now.

Her husband stopped talking to her after treatment started although he would take her to the doctor when the visit was scheduled. No friends to talk to... no time and now even the husband stopped communicating with her.

Kusum started to feel suffocated and restless. Kids were too small to be told anything. They had to be looked after by her. Her mother in law always cribbed that her husband had to spend time and money on her treatment which was a big waste. She had often commented that family would have been better off had Kusum died due to her disease. When a lady has a son she gets some love and respect in the family Kusum thought and here she got nothing. Although Kusum wanted to use contraception she could never communicate that to her husband. She even had to undergo MTP once. Every time her mother in law mouthed bad words about her, Kusum's desire to recover got stronger. She consoled herself by saying she had to live for her kids and soon enough they would be old enough to look after themselves and her. She prays every single day to Almighty that her disease should not come back. She still has to undergo radiation therapy followed by medication for another 5 years and she is prepared to complete the treatment against all odd.

STORY 2

A TEACHER'S LESSON

Anjali loved to teach. Although she was a housewife of 40 years who had enough opportunities to teach her children aged 16 and 12years but still she would teach children of her locality. Money was no constraint. Her husband was financially well off. He was a senior level consultant with a construction company. He travelled often. Anjali would often complaint of being left behind but would teach the children with even more passion. It was their wedding anniversary and she was home with children. She had prepared for the special evening with husband. She prepared a special meal and bought him a gift. Her husband returned that night from Singapore after 5 days. Family was happy to be together in celebrations. He brought gifts for all. It was over dinner that night he promised his family that they would all go for vacation to UAE in winter vacation. His declaration made him the hero for the night... kids were ecstatic and so was Anjali.

It was while they were planning a visit to UAE at the time of getting the visa certain medical tests were required. Doctor suggested that she should have a mammogram also as she was 40 now. So as a screening test mammography was performed. She had dressed up in the morning to go for the tests. She remembered not to apply any deodorant and talcum powder after bathing as instructed by the doctor. She reached the imaging centre and waited for her turn. The scene at the centre was very busy. Women, men, children , those on wheel chairs, beds, white hair, black hair, no hair all were waiting for their turn to get some or the other procedure. Anjali was given a few forms to fill. She did that and started to go through the magazines kept on the nearby table. Attendant at the hospital called Anjali... who is Anjali Singh? 15 years…..and Anjali got up startled when she saw a teenager get up and walk towards the attendant with her mother did she realise that call was not for her but for the teenager.

She was next for an ultrasound to be done in the adjacent room. There were people with water bottle in their hand and were drinking from it while they waited their turn. She wondered why a test with a scheduled appointment took so much of waiting. She changed into a blue gown and was directed to the mammography unit. A lady technician awaited her. Anjali was asked to remove her gown from the upper body and the procedure was explained. Anjali was asked if she had any symptoms related to breast or a family history of any such problem for which her reply was NO. She was instructed to position her breasts one by one in between two plates of the mammography machine. Anjali complied. One plate came from the top and flattened her breast following which X-ray images were taken. Again the breast was repositioned and images were taken. Similarly the procedure was carried out on the other breast. Anjali could feel the discomfort of two metallic plates squeezing and pressing the most sensitive part of her body. She even felt her collar bone being squeezed. She told the technician about it. Technician reassured her that it was required to get good images. After that Anjali was asked to wait in that room till the technician made sure from the radiologist that the images were of good quality or if any other view was to be taken. Anjali waited in that cold room for the technician to return. She had never ever undergone such a procedure in her life and nor had she seen any other woman undergo it. She remembered her mother, mother in law....aunts, no one had ever undergone this test. Technician returned to the room and asked her again if she was sure she had no problem related to breast or had felt a lump. Anjali's reply was again No...She saw the concern on the technician's face and asked her if everything was fine? That is when it was disclosed to Anjali that the radiologist wanted to speak with her and she should change and come out. Anjali was taken to separate room where radiologist was seeing the images on her computer screen. She revealed to Anjali what she was seeing was suggestive of malignancy or cancer.

Anjali was dumbstruck. She asked the doctor to make sure that it was her images only and not that of another patient by the name of Anjali as that name was pretty common. Radiologist confirmed that there was no confusion and it was her test result only. Anjali panicked ...her breathing became fast. She said but "I have no pain or lump in my breast....no problem what so ever...I just came because it was casually suggested by a doctor whatever you are telling me cannot be correct. Had there been any chance of cancer my doctor would have told me".

Radiologist explained to her that patients are diagnosed at the time of screening only and she should get in touch with a hospital to have other investigations done especially biopsy. Anjali called up her husband in a state of panic and told him what the doctor was suspecting. He left his office to be with Anjali.....they scheduled the appointment with doctor and Anjali's stage II cancer was treated. Doctor at the hospital told her that it is very rare that Indian women examine their breasts or go for tests as recommended by the doctor she was lucky that she listened to suggestion of her doctor and went for mammography and the cancer could be detected early. She learnt a new lesson in her life.

STORY 3

STORY OF MY SISTERS

We lived in Meerut not very far away from Delhi. I did my schooling from there. I have a younger and an elder sister. We lived in a huge house and my father worked at the postal department. My mother was a house wife and never been to school. I enjoyed special privilege as I was the only son of the family. Often I would miss school and go and watch a movie. Even if my teachers complained about my irregularity at school my father hardly listened to them. He was confident his son would grow up to be a responsible person. Mother would turn away by saying it was just a passing phase.

During summer vacation my cousins would come from the village to stay with us. They found the television set very fascinating.....we would watch television programmes for hours at a stretch whether they concerned us or not. We would go to mango orchids of my father and spend the day there plucking mangoes and a splash in water. Those times were fun. My elder sister, Saraswati was 16 years and I was about 11 years or 12.

Women from neighbourhood and even people from villages started to visit our home. I had never seen them and was not interested in meeting them other than the fact a lot of sweets and goodies were made available to them to eat so I also got a good share of them. Saraswati *didi* was the quiet and introvert type and recently finished high school. Since women were not encouraged to interact with outsiders and she being the eldest bore the brunt. She would help my mother with household work. My younger sister Urmil was 6 years. I would often tease her and bully her and we landed up fighting almost every day.

One day I saw my father call the local contractor of the area and instructed him to repair the house and white wash it. He was in a hurry to get the house furnished. I did not understand the emergency till one day when my parents were taking Saraswati *didi* to market for shopping did I create a scene and wanted to tag along with them and they refused. They wanted me and Urmil to stay back home.My mother explained to me that Saraswasti *didi's* wedding was fixed and she was to get married in a month's time and shopping had to be done for the bride on urgent basis. She promised me that soon she would take me also to the market to get new clothes.

The house was decked up and foot fall of all types of visitors increased. Saraswati *didi* was married in the following month to a boy who had some agricultural land in a nearby village. My sister moved to the village with him. Time passed I did graduated and found a job with a telecom company in Delhi. It was during those days I heard that Saraswati *didi* had come to stay with my parents as she was not well. No one would tell me the nature of the illness as our family hardly communicated women's problems with men. My sister had been unwell for years but had not said a word to her husband also about it. She grew week and lost a lot of weight and would faint often. No amount of special diet and *desi* treatment helped her in the village that is when her husband left her with my parents to recover .My mother took my sister to a local hospital and further to another one at Lucknow and that is when I came to know that my sister had breast cancer……It was too late and she died within 5 months.

My younger sister wanted to study beyond school and in spite of opposition from my parents she did graduation and B.Ed and started to teach in a school in Meerut. Constant arguments and fights with her parents made her distant and aloof. She would not talk for days. My parents tried to get her married but could not find a suitable and agreeable match as Urmil did not want to meet the same fate as her elder sister and go to a village to live. Urmil is now 35 and I am 41 years old. She teaches and manages the house and my parents are old. Last year Urmil felt a big lump in her breast while taking a bath. She went to a private practitioner. He said she had a fibro adenoma which was anon-cancerous condition and nothing to be worried about. Few months' later pain followed and on visit this time the same doctor gave her a painkiller to be taken. On my visit to my parent's house I enquired Urmil what exactly was going on with and that is when I managed to extract some information from her. I got her to Delhi with me and took her to a lady doctor. She examined her asked for a few investigations. I asked Urmil to stay in Delhi till her investigations were completed. She did not like it here and also my parents were alone in Meerut she agreed to stay...I guess the problem must have bothered her enough and that is why the decision to stay back.

At the clinic I remember the doctor asking me if I had any member in the family who had breast cancer and my response was No......At the time of FNAC also same question was asked, both Urmil and I said that no one had ever had breast cancer in the family. FNAC was inconclusive and so was mammography. But on examination the doctor suspected a cancer I guess, so she sent us to a cancer hospital. We reached there and doctor looked at the reports and examined her .On examination he was quiet sure that the lump was a cancer lump. Biopsy was done and the diagnosis was confirmed. She was operated upon and the breast was removed. I was myself very scared as I did not have much of an exposure to such a treatment and in Meerut we would manage most of the conditions with *desi* treatment. It was after the surgery that doctor had called to plan the rest of the treatment did he ask me again about the family history and this i could not hide it and told him that my elder sister had died of breast cancer. I could see the doctor was both astonished and irritated with me. He asked me why all this while I had hidden this bit of information. I was embarrassed and had no clear reply to give. Somewhere Urmil and I both wanted to bury the health issue of my elder sister and not let it be cause of social stigma. Also I hardly understood the relevance of such a history from doctor's point of view. I kept thinking to myself what held me back from telling the doctors that my elder sister was a victim of breast cancer?

STORY 4

HELP YOUR SELF

Hetal has always been interested in her health. She often lectured her parents and children about healthy eating and exercise. She was 40 years of age and a manager with an airline office. It was in one of the breast awareness workshops that was conducted in her office one year back she learned about many details regarding structure of breast, breast self-exam, mammography, high risk factors and so on.

Hetal observed that both her breasts had gradually over the past 5 months turned painful. She tried to manage herself with a painkiller but that did not help her much. She then decided to talk to a surgeon. Ultrasound of breast showed cysts in both the breasts and her breasts were dense on mammography. Since she had ovarian cysts also she followed up with her gynaecologist. She continued to do breast self-exam every month and was advised to go for mammography and ultrasound every year. She showed her reports to her gynaecologists. Things went on as it is.

In the following year, while doing a self-exam she felt a small tiny thickened area in her left breast at the same spot where she had pain because of the cyst. When she went for the ultrasound it showed nothing new and mammogram also showed the same finding as previous year that of dense breasts. Her gynaecologist asked her not to worry as all was well. In fact she was given anxiolytics to calm her down as nothing new was felt by the doctor. But Hetal was very restless and could not sleep for days she was sure there was something amiss. She followed up with a surgeon next week and he advised fine needle aspiration cytology, which did not reveal anything significant. Again she was sent off with painkillers and advised not to think about it much. She went back grudgingly but was preoccupied with the thought that she and only she could be most familiar with her breasts and if she felt there was a something unusual then that must be correct but how to convince the doctors? Was it just a benign cyst or was there something more to it?

Three months later she felt that the thickened area had developed a small lump. She panicked and discussed the matter with her colleagues at office and they advised her to see the surgeon at once even if her visit was not due. She gathered the courage to fix up an appointment feeling scared at the back of her mind that he might again send her back and label her to be paranoid. How she hated to wait for her turn at doctor's office! There was a big crowd of women with relatives who occupied every nook and corner of the jam packed outpatient department. Some follow up patients after surgery, some on radiation therapy, some having finished chemotherapy and some into remission. All looked stressed with creases on their forehead waiting for their name to be called and given clearance by the doctor that all was clear and they would be normal again or further battery of investigations converting into many more visits to the hospital and many more days of absence from work, borrowing more of money, selling off the property etc. Finally Hetal's turn came to enter the doctor's chamber. She stated her concern to the doctor and he examined her. This time doctor was rather quiet during the examination and asked her more questions about the new development and after that asked for a biopsy. Hetal was petrified now... she knew something was wrong and doctor wanted to confirm that. Her concern was "What if it is a cancer? Must have spread by now...no one listened to me when I came last time. Why is the doctor looking so serious this time"?Following week her biopsy was done and the lump turned out to be a breast cancer....Her world shattered in front of her eyes. Deep down inside she had sensed it ......but felt helpless. It was stage I of the disease and a lumpectomy was performed on her within 2 weeks' time. Admitted in the hospital ward she often thought to herself had she not been so particular about examining herself and keeping track of her abnormal finding in the breast , may be cancer would have been detected much later and her doctors could agree more with her. She insists one should listen to one's own body..... if it does not feel normal, wake up and take charge ,be convinced, you and only you are in the best position to help yourself.

STORY 5

FIGHTER'S STORY

Life has been too busy for Indrani, the eldest daughter of a middle class family. She lost her father when she was barely 2 years. She had taken it upon herself to look after the daily needs of two younger sisters and one brother and old ailing mother, who turned paraplegic due to a stroke two years ago.

She was 44, never married and a senior officer holding a coveted post in a government office, satisfied with herself that in a man's world she could fend for her family members. She was very proud of her achievement.

One day, while getting ready for office she felt a lump of the size of a *kala chana*, about (one cm) in her left breast and when she pressed it there was no pain. She had an urgent meeting to attend so she pushed it to the back of my mind. The lump did not bother her in any way. It remained like that for a year. Although she had heard it should be reported to a doctor, but still did not pay attention. She thought painless lump was nothing serious to be bothered about.

Her only brother started preparing for his twelfth board exams that year and that became the focus of attention for her. If he did well and got a good job, she would prove to be a good sister. She often was hard on herself and side-lined her needs and requirements to prove her worth. Then one day she noticed that the lump had increased in size and the area around it had become hard but she continued to neglect it, forgot all about the lump and life continued getting hectic by the day due to growing responsibilities. Over a few months Indrani noticed that the lump increased in to about size to 4 x 3 cm and now she panicked as something had to done about it proactively.

Breast problem! Now which doctor to go to for consultation, a surgeon? a gynaecologist? Or any nearby lady doctor as it would be most comfortable discussing breast related problem with her. She was so confused. She could not tell anyone at home ....who to talk to who to consult? She could hardly think straight suddenly she remembered Saroj, her friend who suffered from breast cancer. Indrani called her at 2AM and bombarded her with all the pent up questions. Saroj was alarmed at her questions and knew from the tone of her voice that something was not right. She pacified Indrani and promised to take her to the doctor. This is when the hell broke loose. The doctor examined her and asked her for how long the lump had been there. On hearing her answer, he scolded her and told her that she had not behaved like an educated person and had sought the doctor's opinion so late. He wrote CA breast in the case sheet. She thought CA breast could mean breast cancer but her denial instinct came to her rescue and she thought it must be some other medical terminology as breast cancer could not possibly affect her.

She never ever thought in her life that she would get it. She could not understand that it meant breast cancer. Wherever the doctor sent her for investigations everybody helped her on a priority basis without asking any question. Probably they all felt sorry for her. Indrani could not understand the reason for this extra helpful behaviour.

The doctor asked her to arrange for INR 50,000 for surgery. He then told her that he suspected breast cancer but only FNAC (fine needle aspiration cytology) would confirm the diagnosis. Everything changed thereafter. Now, she had to tell her family members about it. Indrani was the strongest of them all. Other family members started to cry. The lump was restricted to one breast and no lymph nodes were involved. Surgery was uneventful.

The doctor told her that this disease was as common as common cold and a person can be treated if it is detected in time. As soon as she started recovering from the surgery, the painful chemotherapy started. This led to a lot of nausea and vomiting and she suffered a lot. Now arose the thought of abandoning treatment and at this point, Indrani preferred death to the intolerable chemotherapy. Saroj and other friends from office came to know of it and they started calling her and counselling her. Her doctor did the best possible for her and her family prayed. Somehow, she completed the treatment.

The side-effects settled down, and she started feeling better. Hair started to grow on her head again and she was reborn. Now, she makes it a point to examine my breasts at home and go to the doctor for follow-up visits. She has been disease-free for twelve years now. She often sits back and thinks what led to so many problems for her — her being the eldest in the family, born as woman, a sensitive part of her body getting affected or the mind-set that teaches that women should sacrifice all for others without taking care of their own needs. Probably, what helped her most were the words of her doctor that "This disease is as common as common cold and can be treated if detected in time."

STORY 6

DANCE WITH LIFE

Salem is a small town located in South India. Gyathri was born there 34 years ago. Her father, Nigur and mother Sachei both were natives of that place. They took pride in promoting art and culture of that place to the rest of the country.

When Gyathri was 3 years old they decided to shift to Delhi in search of greener pasture. Nigur took up the job of a dance teacher in a school and his wife took evening classes for girls and trained them in *Bhartnatyam* form of dance. They rented a small garage in a posh area of south Delhi. Sachei worked as domestic help. The couple had barely finished high school. Nigur on getting exposed to fast paced life of Delhi wanted to get too much too soon and this was developing into a cause of concern as Sachei and Nagur would often get into heated arguments that would often take an ugly turn and Nagur would land up beating his wife after getting drunk. Little Gyathri was growing up amongst this form of domestic violence and chaos. She was admitted in the same school where her dad taught and also the principal waived off her tuition fee as she knew that the family was too poor to support her education in an upmarket south Delhi public school. Gyathri started going to school but it was at primary level of schooling the teachers realised Gyathri could not cope up with her studies, her home work was often not completed and she would miss school on the pretext of some illness or the other. Her parents would fight every night in her presence and it took toll on her emotional wellbeing. Gyathri wanted her parents to be happy and at peace with each other. That was not meant to be.

Nigur got romantically involved with another woman from neighbourhood and would spend nights out with her. Sachei initiallytried probing him about it but it would further lead to fights. Slowly and gradually she accepted this as her fate and learned to keep silent. She started to receive complaints from school about Gyathri but could not help her with studies as she herself had not completed schooling. One day her husband threw her belongings out of the house and asked her to leave them. Poor Sachei had no option but to leave. She moved to another area and started working as domestic help there. In the meantime Gyathri developed an escape mechanism. She would try and run away from home in the evening to play with kids around so that she did not have to witness the daily quarrel and unhappiness in her mother's eyes and now even her loving mother was gone. She became lonelier, sadder and scared…In the process she neglected the school further; she just wanted to be a happy child.

There was an international dance festival to be organized in November that year in Delhi where artists from various countries were expected to participate. Nigur also registered to perform there. It was during this time he met Celia an American artist who was so impressed with Indian dance forms that she decided to stay back in India for a year and learn Indian dance style. Nigur was very impressed with her and at once offered to teach her dance for free. Initially he would teach her thrice a week but slowly they became very fond of each other and would meet every day.

One day Celia told Nagur she wanted to move in with him and live with him. She offered to hire a room for them to stay. Since both of them loved each other they started staying together Gyathri had to stay with them. Gyathri could barely understand why her father started to stay with Celia. Gyathri would often go to school without breakfast and lunch box and would eat other's lunch. She was sad. During this time she came to know Mir ,a tailor who worked in the local market. He was 17 years of age. He would chat with her in the evenings. She told him the details of her family situation. This boy often hung around with bigger boys who would drink and pass comments on girls at the market place. One evening, while she was returning home one of the boys told her that Mir wanted to speak with her. She accompanied him. He took her to the garage where he stayed and raped her. That was a dark gory night in the life of Gyathri. She was a sad girl but now wanted to die…

She came home and shutoff completely from the outside world .She did not say a word about this to her father or else he would beat her up and lock her inside the house. In the meantime her father and his girlfriend had a baby boy and all the attention was focused on the newborn. Gyathri just wanted to leave this world and disappear. She had often heard from Celia about life in

USA and wanted to go off to this foreign land and start a life there.

She once told her father about it and he thought of sending her away. He borrowed some money and made arrangements for her to leave the country. Gyathri was all of 16 all alone when she reached Florida.

She got in touch with Indian cultural associations whose address she had carried and started to teach dance over there. She would even model par time to make a living .All her time was spent in making a living but she was happier somehow. She made friends. All in all liked the foreign land and the breathing space it provided her.

Two years later Nigur married Celia and they also decided to move to USA. Since they did not tell Gyathri about it she had no news of them. She wanted to forget the past.

Gyathri learned other dance forms and obtained proficiency in them. She moved to Washington and hired a small flat .It was then she met this boy from Iraq Zahir, who had come to do graduation there. No doubt he was from a very rich business family based in Iraq. They became good friends. They wanted to get married but both knew how his family would respond to a Hindu girl from India so they decided to get married in Washington itself. Everything was dreamlike. They were madly in love with each other and a year later Amir was born.

After 2 years Zaheer had to return home to Iraq so Gyathri gave up her career and stared to pack everything. All she wanted was to be happy in life with a family she could call her own which was denied to her during childhood.

In Iraq, Zahir got a warm welcome from his family. His mother, father, elder brother his wife and elder sister rejoiced at his arrival. He joined the family business of leather upholstery and soon expanded their export to Africa and other Asia countries. Zahir would travel often and was totally engrossed in work but for Gyathri after the initial euphoria settled things were going to be very different. Her mother in law and Zahir's elder sister would often tease her about her small frame. They would not let her enter the prayer room. One day things took an ugly turn. Gyathri's mother in law took Amir away from her told her that she converted to Islam they would not let her near him. Gyathri in order to hold on to her happiness agreed to everything her mother in law said. Gyathri was sent to another city in a rural area for one year in their ancestral home. She was to say there and learn all about Islam and Quran. Gyathri could not bear the pain of separation from her son and cried every single day. She fasted for days and months and would eat very little and tried to focus on learning as many religious scripts as possible.

After one year when she returned home her mother in law questioned her about her learning and only then gave Gyathri permission to stay with them .Still things did not improve. One day Gyathri was told that her mother in law wanted to keep Amir and did not want her in the family. Since nothing improved the situation Gyathri thought of returning to Washington but not without her son. She told Zahir if he ever loved her he would let her go back with her son. Zahir who still loved her agreed to it and could not bear to see Gyathri suffer so much. But he did not have the guts to move out due to a combined family business. Gyathri came back and started to live by herself.

She tried to put her life back on the track. She gradually started with the dance practice and joined a school as a teacher. It was during that time while trying on a well fitted dress for a dance performance that she felt she had a lump in her left breast. She was terrified ....she knew it could be a cancer and that involved a body mutilating surgery. She focussed on the work at hand and following week took and appointment to see a doctor. Investigations confirmed her hidden fear. Gyathri had stage II breast cancer and was in need of surgery. She refused to undergo mastectomy and no amount of counselling helped. Gyathri did not want to disfigure her body as she believed it would affect her dance and of course she was petrified too. Finally one night she decided that if she wanted to live and get her son back she should listen to the experts. Volunteers helped her with chemotherapy and radiation therapy. They would accompany her to the hospital and even do grocery shopping for her. She now volunteers in her area to help breast cancer patients with treatment and follow ups.

Two years later Gyathri met Wilson, a businessman at a charitable dance performance. He instantly liked

Gyathri and in spite of apprehensions and fears managed to convince her to marry him. Cancer and sadness both have disappeared from Gyathri's life. This is the story of Gyathri's dance with life.

STORY 7

MOTHER WHO COULDNOT BE A ROLE MODEL

My parents have fought since I was very young, since I was in kindergarten to be specific. At the start, it was very bad. There would be endless screaming and shouting and physical abuse sometimes. He and mom fought often. When I was in class 6th I remember, once I got low grades in Maths and English that is when my dad got furious and beat me up black and blue.....ever since I stayed away from him. Before he came home at night I would pretend I was asleep. Listened to constant arguments and fights every night......finally one day they decided to get divorced and I was so glad that we all would lead a happy life even if it meant separately.

My mother decided to send me to a boarding school. I was sent to Dehradun to study. I realised early in life that I had to study hard and make a good career and become financially independent so that I could have my say and my say alone in my matters. I would only come home during vacation and meet my father once in a while. My mom made it a point to make my vacation special. I graduated from a law school and joined the high court and started to enjoy working there. In the meantime my mom retired from service and went to stay with her brother at Kolkata.

It was during a visit to Kolkata in May, last year back when courts were closed while talking to my mom I realised she had lost a lot of weight and looked very frail. On my enquiring about her diet she would say all was well and that she was eating well. Somehow, I was not convinced and kept probing her. Finally she told me that blood was coming out of her breast for the past couple of days and she had been having fever and once fever subsides all would be fine. She had not bothered to consult any physician. I was concerned and booked an appointment with the doctor next day. On examining the breasts doctor asked for how many days the problem was going on and had she got any investigation done. After doing a complete physical check-up he hinted that my mother could be having breast cancer and that investigations were required. Within a week all the tests were done and diagnosis was confirmed. It was a stage III breast cancer. Surgery was done and after a gap of few days chemotherapy would begin.

Glimpses of my mother how she took care of me and my father when we fell sick often pass my mind. If I ever had slightest of fever or cold she would take a leave and stay home with me serving me fresh soup and juice and porridge. She would sleep besides me and at night on multiple occasions touch to feel if my fever had settled down. In spite of quarrels with my father she was always besides him if he ever fell sick. She would give in to his whims and fancies and cook whatever he would demand from her. She would even feed him on bed and give medicines with her own hand. I wonder how a lady who stood up for herself and very boldly and single handily looked after her daughter did not bother to look after her health and neglected it. What if parents emphasised as much about health as they did about marriage and children to their daughters? Awareness about health issues is the way forward and parents should be role models.

STORY 8

TRUTH OF MANY A WOMEN

Nisha had been married to Satya for over two decades now. They had a very happy and fulfilling married life till now. Elder son had finally entered college and the daughter had completed graduation, a signal for Nisha and Satya to look for a prospective groom for her daughter and get her settled in the near future. Nisha had been the back bone of the family. Every morning she would get up at 4.30 am prepare breakfast and lunch for all, followed by morning tea and then wake them up. She would fetch the newspaper as and when it arrived and hand it to her father in law lest he might feel disconnected from the world. And waiting impatiently ask again and again *"Bahu paper aya kya?"*. Even her mother in law! Had never raised and doubt about the competency of Nisha in handling the home turf. Nisha herself was a graduate but took pride in being a homemaker as her in laws and husband wanted a girl who would manage the house well rather than stepping put in man's world. Satya who was a professor in university also somewhere deep down in his heart was comfortable with the idea of his being the sole bread winner for the family and hence had carried an air of superiority. Living in Delhi it is an uphill and daunting task for couples to get their child to finish schooling and enter college. It requires years of preparation, extra classes, tuitions, numerous trips to examination centres and so on. For Nisha and Satya it was no different. For about 2 years at least the whole family has to lead a disciplined life as they did not want their child's 12th class grades and chances of getting admission into a good college dwindle.

It was while the son was preparing for his 11th standard exam did Nisha feel heaviness in the chest for first time. She was not sure if actually felt something different .After about 2 months she felt a hard area in her breast. She now was sure something was abnormal but ...."Let it be" was her response. When her son reached final of school one day while cooking she again felt some heaviness in her left breast and when she touched it there was a definite lump. She pressed it.... it caused some discomfort but did not hurt. Now she thought maybe she should tell her husband about it but time passed. She over a period of time lost appetite and felt weak and insisted her daughter help her with household chores which in a way would also prepare her for marriage. Her daughter suspected something was not right with her mother and insisted that she be taken to hospital for consultation. That week at the hospital the general physician realised that Nisha was not well at all sent her to a surgeon. That is when the detailed investigations were done and it was found that she on mammography and confirmed on biopsy that she had breast cancer. She was already in stage IIIs of the disease which is an advanced stage of the disease.

What happened after that no one could have imagined. Satya had to come with his wife to the hospital every day. She was operated and then chemotherapy was started. It was during the second cycle of chemotherapy she felt she could not take it any, more the nausea and the weakness and dependency on others in the family. She did not want to continue with the treatment but doctors called her to complete the chemo therapy. This was to be followed by one month of ordeal of radiation therapy too. Nisha's husband took her for radiation therapy for two days when she insisted that now she would be fine and did not need treatment any more. The husband tired of all the running around himself thought she had been under treatment for too long and must be actually feeling normal. They did not bother to go for radiation therapy after that and Nisha after some time tried getting back to her daily schedule with much effort but she was not going to be herself again. Due to weakness one night she fainted on the floor on her way to the washroom. Satya was woken up from his sleep by a loud noise. He looked around to see and saw that his wife was missing from the bed besides him. He looked further and found Nisha lying on the floor, unconscious. He rushed her to the hospital. Her soul had left the body. Doctors declared her dead. Nisha died due to complications of breast cancer in stage IV. Nisha had neglected her health and took two years to visit a doctor and had not completed the treatment. Satya married again one year later. This is the truth of many a women.

STORY 9

FOR OTHERS IT IS LIKE A STORY

Rashmi had started to enjoy her life again after a painful divorce. She was a religious person. She performed *pujas* and fasted on auspicious days every month. She was a social worker by profession and earned enough to sustain her. She was fond of watching movies with friends and help all those in need to an extent possible by her.

It all started in Sept 2002, when she felt a pain in the left breast and along with that also a small lump. Following which she started going to a general surgeon of a hospital as she was not very confident of doing breast self-examination. The doctor started her on hormones and she kept on going for regular check-ups, according to him it was normal for age and nothing to worry about and that a lot of women come to him with these kind of problems. He prescribed me Vitamin E and some other medicine. Rashmi took all the prescribed medicines. Couple of times he also suggested FNAC and some other investigations as well. The reports turned out to be negative for cancer. Every time she went for FNAC the experience was excruciating as doctors had a difficult time putting the needle into the breast for FNAC. They would find it difficult to target the lump. It went on for two years and all the reports turned out to be negative. Then one day Rashmi thought of taking a second opinion from the same hospital. Immediately on seeing me, this time the doctor suggested a mammogram. And the radiologist while doing mammography told her that what he was seeing was not good. He said that if "she wanted to live, she should get an ultrasound guided FNAC next day". Rashmi got very disturbed on listening to this. The next day sample was taken and in the evening she was told on phone that it was cancer of breast. Just imagine it started with one lump and it increased to 6. In two years' time the lump increased from one to six in number and she could feel it all. Although only one was malignant out of these six. She was surprised that even on her insistence of getting a mammogram done; the doctor kept saying that there was no need for a mammogram and in fact discouraged her from getting it done and said everything will be fine. And here now she was with CANCER !

Rashmi had been a strong person all her life but at this moment felt very weak and vulnerable. She would cry the whole night and thought of spending the rest of her life visiting a hospital disturbed her the most. Images of taking appointments and visiting hospital for her entire life came to her .She thought follow ups won't be easy either. She would never live her life as a free person without the burden of this disease weighing on her mind. No more carefree vacations.....no more carefree celebrations.....and the bank balance had to look good too. Her mother and relatives thought that the world has come to an end, everything was over for her.

Finally surgery was done followed by chemotherapy which started after 21 days at a premier cancer hospital of Delhi. By the grace of God she had no problem with the treatment in the sense that the operating surgeon was very cooperative. So he went ahead with the surgery. Axillary lymph nodes were also taken out. Out of 18, 8 were malignant. The cost involved was Rs. 45,000.Chemotherapy started exactly 21 days after surgery. Chemotherapy drugs itself cost her INR 75,000 and after first cycle she had febrile neutropenia. Hurriedly she was admitted .TLC was very low. This admission amounted to INR 35,000. So approximately one hundred and ten thousand was the money spent for one cycle and for six cycles of chemotherapy her expected expenditure was going to be close to seven hundred thousand of INR! She could feel the financial crunch. Her family supported her with money as they wished the best for her. Chemotherapy was very painful. In her word, "drugs are like poison and it is poison kills poison." She could not eat or drink anything all the time she had nausea, vomiting, pain in abdomen, you lost your taste buds, and very big mouth ulcers. Rest other superficial things like hair fall and pigmentation also happened. Rashmi was completely shattered. She had to wear mask all the time. Life became very restricted. At times she felt during the chemotherapy that she should stop the treatment and let myself die since one has to die anyway one day.

When she was operated she was told a swelling of the arm could arise but nothing happened for one year. Two years later all of a sudden a swelling started in her left arm, the side on which operation was done, it kept increasing slowly. She consulted the cancer surgeon, who prescribed antibiotics and pressure garment, both all these did not help. Now she felt like a handicap who could only work with one hand. She needed another huge amount for the lymph drainage pump. Resources just kept getting thinner and thinner by the day. She had heard one has to go for follow up to the doctor once in 3 months' time but in her case in a week at least one to two days she still have to spend in the OPD as something or the other issue kept cropping up. She does not want to repeat the same mistake of relying on one doctor and neglect herself anymore.

She often tells her friends "One a lady, second a disease in a very sensitive part of her body, she detects the disease in very early stage but the doctor cannot perform his duty perfectly. Not only the lady but her whole family suffers from the problems. Lot of money is spent. Is it needed that some special training needed to be imparted to doctors for treating breast lumps effectively? May be doctor are preoccupied with too many patients or do not have enough experience but they should never take the complaints of the patients casually." She was not confident of examining her breasts she did not know how to do it and felt guilty for that. Rashmi believes that a patient is never wrong it is the doctor who is not able to understand the patient's complaints; maybe it is the limitation of their subject. Whatever the patient is saying she a problem there has some basis or the other. One does not complain for no reason. Patient for her safety should go to more than one doctor for opinion. Only a person who has gone through the misery can describe and nobody else. For others it's like a story.

STORY 10

MOVE ON

Preeti was a quiet and an introvert girl. She was born in the city of Indore. Right from her birth in a city hospital till graduation she had stayed there only. She had a few college and school friends, all girls with whom she would go out occasionally to picnic. It was after she got married that she moved to Delhi. She was 28 years at that time. She found Delhi to be too big a place to live. She thought to herself if ever she got lost on the roads she would never be able to reach back home by herself. She and her husband Sahil both worked for the same bank. It was a big relief for her that at least she did not have to commute by herself as their office was 20 kilometres away from their residence. In the morning and evening on their drive back home he would show her different buildings and land marks. They would at times stop midway to have corn or ice cream. They were trying to bond and get to know each other better as it was an arranged marriage for them. Sahil tried to make Preeti as comfortable as possible and tried to make her get accustomed to crazy ways of a big metropolitan city. Sahil's parents and younger brother stayed with them.

The young couple was new to the job, so were trying to consolidate their career and have a healthy bank balance. They had no plans of starting the family at least for the next 2 years. Preeti's mother in law was a doctor at a private hospital. She did not interfere much in their lives and wanted the young couple to be happy. Almost two years had passed it was during that time that Preeti complained of feeling weak and fatigued. She also revealed she felt heaviness in the breasts. Initially she attributed it to the oral contraceptive pills she had started to use. But over the months heaviness and discomfort ion the breast increased and she was taken to a hospital. She was prescribed some vitamins and iron and asked to improve her diet as her haemoglobin was 10gm%.She followed the instructions but did not feel much of improvement. She would go to work in the morning and come back drained out in the evening with no appetite for food. Sahil got worried. He booked an appointment with a doctor at a renowned hospital. There she was examined physically to rule out any major health concerns and was also advised breast ultrasound and if need be a mammogram as she was young for a mammogram. Ultrasound revealed nothing much other than a fatty axillary tail. It was followed by a mammogram. Now, there were a few specks which demanded further probe. It was decided to do a biopsy of the area and histopathology revealed DCIS or the Ductal Carcinoma in Situ. Treating physician was himself shocked that at the age of 30 he was seeing a patient of breast cancer. Although it is considered to be stage 0 but in her case it had a high probability of becoming invasive in spreading.

Everyone was in denial Preeti, Sahil and his parents. "It cannot be a cancer at his age" was there common opinion. No one in her family had breast cancer then how come? They took another opinion and another even flew to Mumbai to meet the oncology experts but the result was the same. Finally, reality set in and the parents decided to start praying. *Havans* and *pujas* were conducted for Preeti's good health. Lumpectomy was performed in Mumbai.

Doctors decided to give her radiation therapy after that. Preeti often thought to herself that she had not even started her family and may be now will never be able to have any children or may not be will not even be there to look after them. Preeti did not want to have radiation therapy for fear of side effects .She thought it might interfere with her chances of conceiving.

Family would console each other but atmosphere at home was glum. Sahil investigated about the alternative medicine practitioners in cancer and discussed Preeti's case with them as it is believed their medicines cause less of side effects. They even went to hills to consult Tibetan practitioners. More of *Pujas* were held case was discussed with anyone with a remote possibility of helping them out.

Alternative therapy was started after surgery but Sahil insisted that Preeti started with radiation therapy as he did not want her to take any chances with her life. Radiation was given in a hospital in Delhi and then Preeti was put on Tomoxifen for 5 years .What it meant was that she won't be able to conceive for the next 5 years or more.

Amidst gloom and pain and tears but with a determination to move on in life the couple decided to adopt a child.

STORY 11

AGENTS OF CHANGE

Sunil Khera was a strict disciplinarian. He was a principal at a government run school in south Delhi. He had the wide experience of working in other states of the country. He believed that discipline had to come from teachers. If teachers set an example then only students could be disciplined. There were two shifts in his school and he was on his toes from morning six to evening seven. It was a co-educational school from first to 12th standard and often there were issues with the senior boys.

On a rainy Saturday morning Raksha walked briskly towards the principal desk she had a very worrisome expression on her face as if something troubled her internally. She portrayed a sense of urgency and could not wait to talk to the principal. She apologised to the principal for coming late to school and requested him not to deduct half day leave for her as was the norm in that school. When the principal inquired what the matter was she started to speak. "Sir, the transfer form does not have a column for separated or divorced women, so in which column should I tick the response while seeking transfer. The marital status column either says married or widow or unmarried? Sir, my transfer application is getting delayed I want my application to be approved at the earliest." Principal looked up from his reading glasses and enquired, " Raksha, have you have not been able to send that man behind bars? He has troubled you so much?"Raksha replied "no sir, they are too smart .They have managed to evade arrest. I only want a quick divorce now." She began to cry. "My husband and in-laws tortured me no end. Gave me physical and mental sufferings I cannot tolerate it any more. I just want things to be normal after my divorce."

Principal acknowledged that the transfer form needed a revision. That day in the school a special programme was organised on breast cancer for the women staff and that was about to start. Principal asked Raksha to go and participate in that health programme. There were 69 teachers in all for the programme. Many were shy to even interact on breast related issues. If any question was asked by a participant others would simply add on a hypothetical question to that and this way without divulging their own issues sought clarification to their concerns .In spite of it being a all women gathering teachers would look away and not meet the gaze of the doctor or else they would be asked something.

In this kind of atmosphere there was one person who would ask a question every 5 minutes and would repeat what was told to her so that she was absolutely sure she had learned the right thing. That person was Raksha. She kept saying she had to take good care of her health as she could not afford to fall ill as she had too many problems on the domestic front to handle. Throughout the programme she was very fidgety and anxious .Those sitting around her looked at her with a sense of amusement, as they found her too restless and too attentive.

At the end of the programme, many were relieved that the ordeal was over, many were thankful for the important issues discussed and many just rushed out to prepare for next class. But one person waited till the room was vacant and spoke with the doctor at length as to how and when she should examine her breasts. She kept saying she was too busy to fall ill.

It was in the following week Raksha decided to examine her breasts after her periods. She felt the breast to be lumpy. She had never examined her breast before this and it was her first exam. She found the breasts to be lumpy but that was expected as told to her in the workshop at school but there was a lump in the right breast which felt a little different from others. She was unsure what it was she got jittery and thought of consulting a doctor.

Whose help to take and where to go? Raksha lived alone in a rented room. She married four years back after two years of courtship. But problems started soon after first year of marriage. Her husband and mother in law started beating her up and wanted to take away all her salary. She resisted as she wanted to save some money for future but the conservative Haryana family she was married into, there was no scope of a lady having her own salary. Her husband now threatened to get her killed. That is why she wanted to move to another city as her life was in danger. Raksha's parents were against her marriage and they cut off all connections with her after marriage. Her mother was a heart patient and father blind from one eye. She was their only child and she had let them down. They could not believe that such a simple and intelligent daughter of theirs could fall for a goon.

Raksha went to a doctor in the nearby hospital where they performed fine needle aspiration and Raksha was in intolerable pain for the next 10 days. That is the time she thought of consulting the doctor had come to their school for the workshop. Raksha was referred to a premier hospital of Delhi where mammography confirmed she had breast cancer. Her breast cancer was in stage II and was to be operated soon. Doctor was glad that she came to the hospital without delay. Now she needed an escort to come to the hospital with her as treatment was going to be long. She informed the school principal and applied for leave. Other teachers came to know of her problem but did not come forward to help her as most of them stayed away from her and avoided her ever since Raksha started to live alone. Even Raksha was not comfortable approaching them.

The thought of talking to her parents crossed her mind but her mother's heart ailment discouraged her from telling them the truth. She felt guilty about wrong marriage, breaking relationship with her parents and now landing up in this new problem. How could she give them more stress?

One night while crying and thinking to herself she made the decision to go to her parents. Once they came to know of her illness they accepted her with open arms and asked her stay with them. Her father accompanied her for the treatment to the hospital. Chemotherapy and radiation therapy followed surgery. Now she is living happily with her parents. She is thankful to the almighty that her disease has brought her close to her parents. Raksha believes women should themselves become agents of change.

www.ingramcontent.com/pod-product-compliance
Lightning Source LLC
Chambersburg PA
CBHW032342200526
45163CB00018BA/2141